REGA

Regan MOVES is gentle and effective.

"Regan MOVES" has two meanings:

- Exercise for QUALITY of life—to have a healthy, meaningful life.
- Exercise for ALL your life—You should be able to do at age 90 what you're doing now. It's all about sustainability and longevity.

This is so exciting! My hope—the reason I'm doing this—is for you to perform Regan MOVES well and feel better. This is the start of your journey towards feeling more capable, powerful, and whole. And by leading by example you will help others.

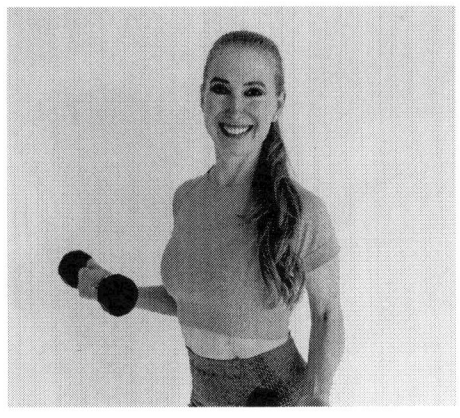

Regan Birr, B.Sc. Mechanical Engineering and Certified Personal Trainer

DISCLAIMER

This book is written as a source of information only. It should not be considered a substitute for the advice of a qualified medical professional. Always consult your doctor before you begin any new diet, exercise, or other health program.

We've made every effort to be sure we have accurate information in this book as of the date published. The author and publisher disclaim responsibility for any adverse effects arising from the use or application of the information contained here.

©2024 Regan Birr

All rights reserved. No portion of this book may be reproduced or stored in a retrieval system in any form or by any means, except for brief quotations in reviews or articles, without the prior written permission of Regan Birr.

Website: ReganMoves.com
Email: regan@reganmoves.com

Cover and interior design by Sharon Brodin, Brodin Press LLC
Photographs by Sara Noel Lee Photography

Regan MOVES™ and JointSense™ by Regan MOVES
© Regan Birr

"Methods to Help Fight the Effects of Chronic Fatigue and Pain"
© Regan Birr, Regan MOVES LLC. All Rights Reserved.

Table of Contents

Introduction
5

What is Regan MOVES and How Can It Help You?
7

Keys to Making It a Calorie-Burner
21

Regan MOVES Exercise Routine Synopsis
25

Regan MOVES Exercise Routine with Detailed Descriptions and Modifications
27

Recap
65

Regan MOVES Levels
67

Regan's Story
69

Regan MOVES Summary
71

Regan MOVES Services
73

Endorsements & Testimonials
75

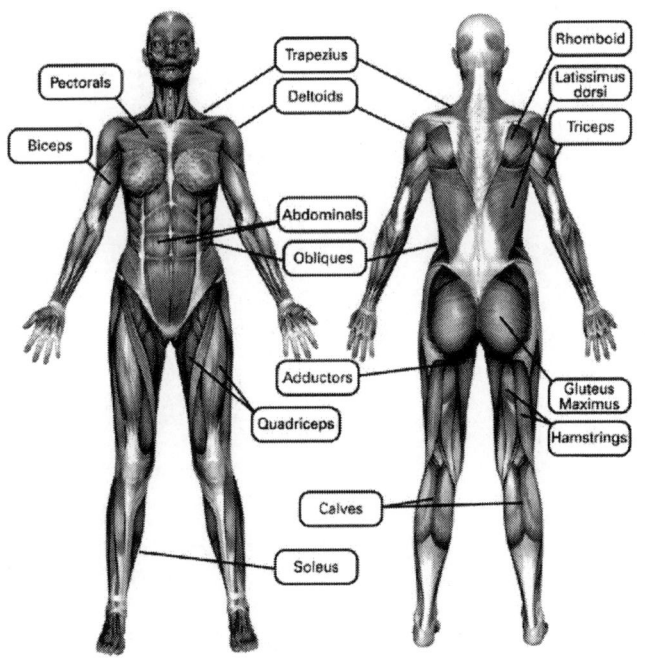

Muscles of the body

Introduction

Regan MOVES is both a noun and a verb. When I was diagnosed with systemic lupus, arthritis, and fibromyalgia I had to MOVE to get my life back. I "Regan MOVED." And of course, it's also a program. Hopefully, the only program you'll ever need.

The premise behind Regan MOVES is to provide low-torque sensible moves for sensitive joints and muscles. There's been much study about how important it is to move when we have pain. The same goes for those of us with lupus, fibromyalgia, and joint injury, as well as mental and emotional health concerns. Everyone should be exercising! This provides a way to do it.

Regan MOVES is a method of movement that empowers you, reminding you that you can work out, achieve energy, and have a normal, happy life. Rediscover the joy of exercise, of movement, and creating a life that is vibrant.

The goal of Regan MOVES is to help you reach vitality and to share your confidence with others. Strengthen the muscles that support the joints and move again. Your joy will spread like a wave of awareness—awareness that everyone can exercise.

This is a movement for *movement*.

Regan MOVES is also designed for people in the general population who simply don't want to put added stress on their knees or other joints. It provides a way to work out safely, more gently, and without discomfort—more aptly, *with* comfort!

Regan MOVES helps reduce the pressure points on the knees, hips, and other joints of the body. And it just makes sense. Regan MOVES makes good sense for your joints.

We all have aches and pains: from instructors to first-time exercisers with chronic conditions. Everybody has something.

The basic thing to remember is that Regan MOVES is low-torque. That means it reduces the distance of the weight from the joint of concern, which results in increased comfort while you work out.

Let Regan MOVES increase your energy and decrease your pain!

What is Regan MOVES and How Can It Help You?

Regan MOVES is:
- A low-torque, low-impact, full body workout
- Joint-safe

Our motto is: "Work smarter, not harder."

"You get a cardio AND strength workout, without the impact or torque."

~ Colleen, lupus patient and Regan MOVER

> The hardest part of getting moving is getting started!
> This program gives you the START you need.

Regan MOVES is: A full-body, gentle-on-your-joints workout with:
- Strength-building segments (low-torque, low-impact)
- Cardio segments (low-torque, low-impact)

Where we:
- Stretch between each segment (optional)
- Create the Challenge constantly (keep our heart rates up the entire time)*

See "Keys to Making It a Calorie-Burner" on p. 21

It's gentle and you do it at your own pace.

The purpose of alternating the segments is to prevent fatigue. It prevents overall fatigue and specifically fatigue of your muscles and joints. It keeps you energized so you are able to keep going and complete the workout. Try it! You'll see.

The purpose of stretching between segments is to keep you in comfort the whole workout.

The goal is to prevent pain and keep you fluid and mobile with increased comfort.

Overview

Regan MOVES is a low-torque exercise program that is geared towards people with chronic conditions and challenges.

Which means it's safe for all people!

Don't let "with chronic conditions" fool you. It doesn't mean the exercises require little effort. It means they're smart. They are gentle on the joints but will challenge you. Besides, people with chronic conditions are tough.

Secondly, this program gets the heart rate up. As high as you want it! The intensity is up to YOU. All while we work smarter, not harder, on the joints. We work *smarter-on-the-joints*.

And everything is customizable. It is gentle, for those with fatigue and pain, to more intense.

It's the perfect system.

Let this be the only exercise program you need!

Everybody knows the positive impact of exercise. Exercise strengthens your joints, lubricates your joints, and helps maintain joint motion and function. It helps you feel better. And it can help you lose weight.

The problem: How do you exercise when you're in pain? Or you're fatigued?

Remember: We're all in the Same Boat and It's OK. You Can Do It. 50 million Americans suffer from arthritis (source: Centers for Disease Control and Prevention). Approximately 1.5 million Americans suffer from lupus.

I suffer from both. And I understand you have challenges too.

History: The first time I tried exercising I cried. The pain was unbearable. I couldn't squat.

The solution: I needed to reduce the torque. I recovered by developing (and sticking to) a low-torque exercise program.

The payoff was huge!
Exercise REALLY improved my life.

What is torque?

> TORQUE is a measure of how much a force acting on an object causes that object to rotate *about an axis*.

Torque is: Force x Distance. Where force is weight, distance is lever. So torque = weight x lever. So, to reduce torque either decrease your force (weight), or decrease distance (your lever).

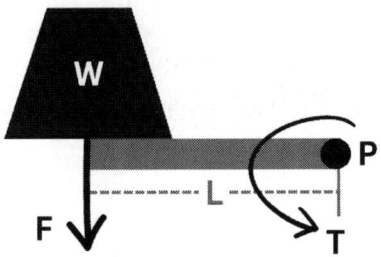

Example 1: T = F x L

Why does reducing torque help us? It reduces pressure points!

> Pressure points on your joints are created when you have torque about your joints.

How to Reduce Torque on Knees

There are two ways to lower the torque:
Reduce your weight
and/or
Reduce your lever

Don't do lunges—or keep your lunge steps small. Small steps equal a smaller lever.

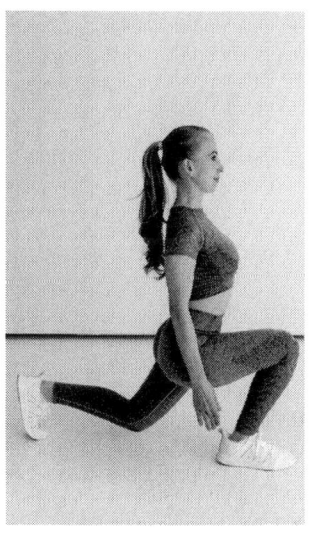 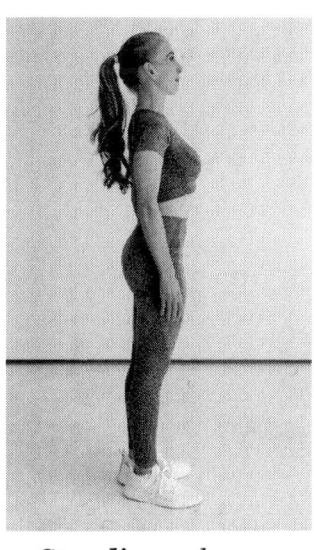

Lunges *add torque and pressure points to the knee*

Standing *reduces or eliminates torque on the knee and distributes weight evenly across the knee joint*

Note: Maybe you *can* do lunges. Just keep the range of motion (ROM) smaller! Work your way up to bigger

ROM. It's up to you. Or just lift up your heel (go up on your toes) to isolate the other leg. Whatever you do, start with a low ROM.

How to Reduce Torque on Shoulders

To lower the torque on shoulders, reduce the weight or reduce the lever. And keep weights over the shoulders, or under the shoulders if you're doing a pull.

(NOTE: Weight refers to either the weight of your arms or free weights.)

When arms are extended up and not directly over the joint, the weight of the arms creates a rotation about the joint (torque):

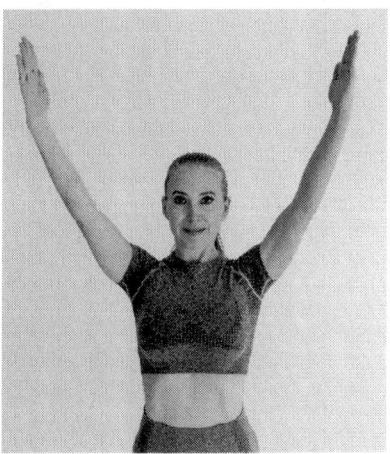

When arms are above the joint (as seen on facing page in two planes), torque is reduced or eliminated.

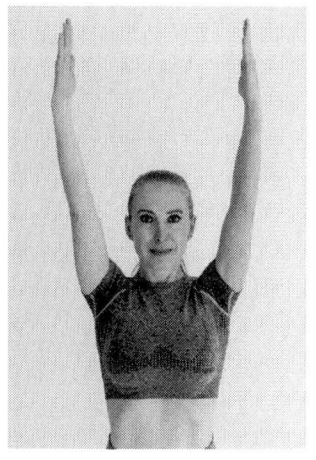 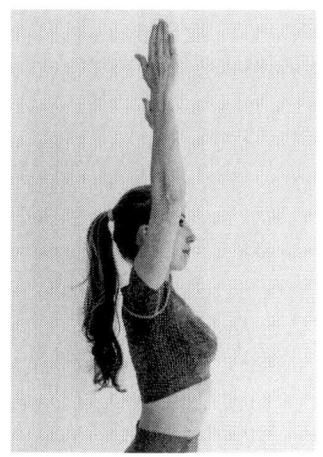

Similarly, when arms are extended in front of you from the shoulder joint, they create rotation about the joint (torque pulls the arms down):

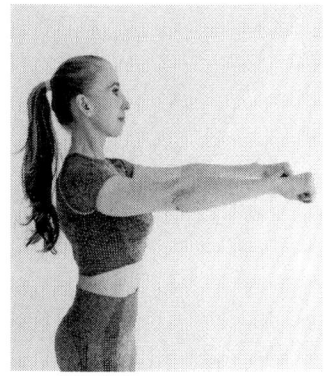 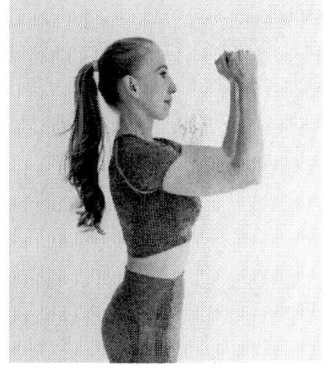

To reduce the torque, simply reduce the lever—bend your arms.

As seen from the front plane, torque pulls (rotates) arms down laterally:

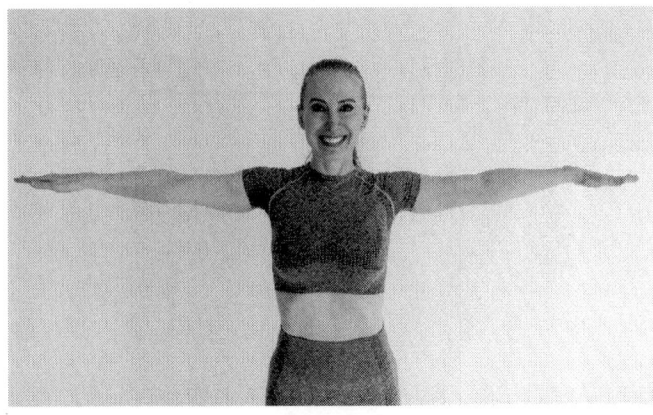

To reduce torque, reduce your lever:

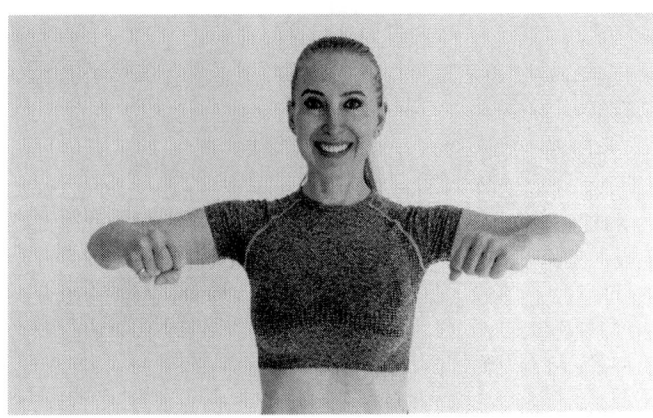

How To Properly Perform a Regan MOVES Squat

> This is extremely important as the Regan MOVES squat is an integral part of the exercises.

The hip bones must be "up and out" such that you look like a skier in an athletic position, ready to attack the slopes.

Keep your squats shallow (to a comfortable depth). Protect your back by keeping it flat or slightly arched, but not rounded. Draw your belly button to your spine. (Note: You can pulse instead of holding squats. This seems to relieve pressure on the knee joints and prevent fatigue.)

This benefits you by incorporating the large muscles, which gets the heart rate up. Large muscles include the glutes, hamstrings, and quads.

It also is extremely valuable in strengthening the muscles that support your knees.

With all movements, keep your arms and legs within the frame of the body.

> **TIP:** A great way to get your heart rate up is to use your large muscles and get your arms over your head. That is why it's important we get this critical movement down pat.
>
> (More on getting your heart rate up in "Keys to Making It a Calorie-Burner" on p. 21.)

Hip bones should be "up" and "out" while your back is safely supported (keep it arched or flat, not rounded, and draw your belly button to your spine):

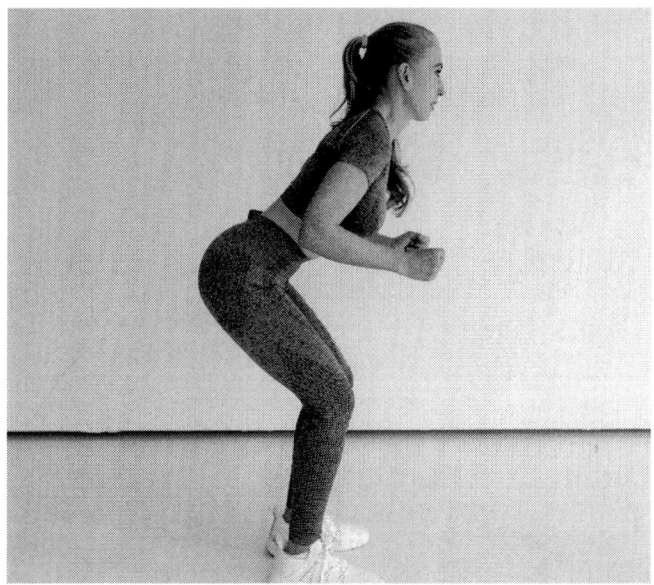

> This is the proper Regan Moves squat. It moves the center of gravity closer to directly above the knees. This decreases torque and increases comfort on your knees.

Do not have your Center of Gravity "behind" your knees:

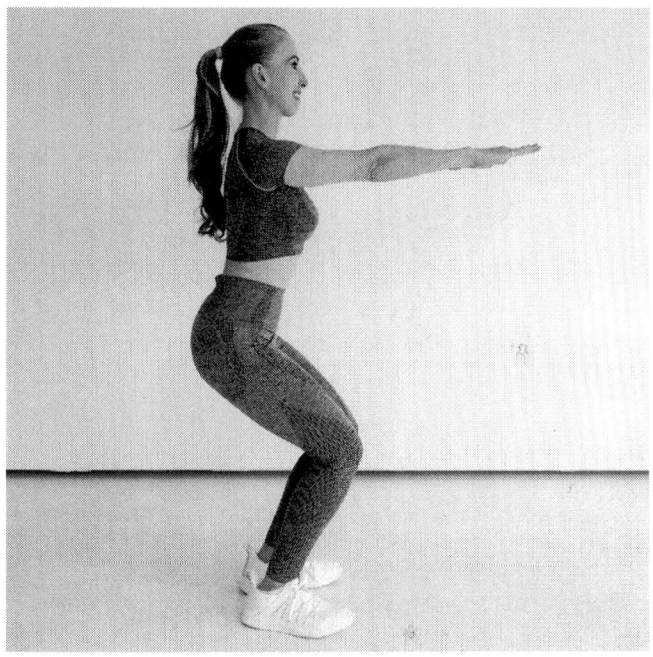

We do not want to have our weight behind our knees as shown above. This puts a tremendous amount of torque on the knees. It feels entirely different from the Regan MOVES "knee-friendly" position.

Summary to Reduce the Torque

To decrease torque we want to reduce the distance of the weight from the joint of concern. (Weight being either the free weights and/or your Center of Gravity (C of G), which is also affected by free weights).

Aim to keep your C of G over the joint that hurts. For example, do not perform lunges. Instead, keep your body weight over the knees and do a shallow squat. This will still work the muscles while reducing the torque on the knees.

Similarly, during a shoulder press, keep weight over your shoulders with your arms as close as possible to directly above your shoulders. This will reduce the torque on your shoulders.

Regan MOVES is about reducing torque.

> Regan MOVES is as much about what you **don't** do as it is about what you do.

Regan MOVES "Do's"

- Keep weight close to the body
- Keep your weight over the joint that hurts
- Keep your limbs within the frame of the body (close to the body)

Examples of torque-filled movements we *avoid* in Regan MOVES:

Lunges—See comprehensive exercise descriptions for ways to isolate each leg as an alternative to lunges. We do RM (specialized) squats instead.

Deep squats—See comprehensive exercise descriptions for modifications of squats that are performed safely without exacerbating pressure points on the knees.

Wide-legged stances as in some yoga poses.

Overhead movements where weights are not held above the shoulder.

Outside-of-the-body movements when arms are held away from the body.

Keys to Making It a Calorie-Burner

The following are keys to keeping your heart rate up during the entire workout.

Create the challenge:

You're going to the effort of working out. So you might as well make it worthwhile, right? To burn calories and lose weight, you'll need to keep your heart rate up.

Not crazy high, just the right amount. And you'll know what this means for you. Every exercise is adjustable, so you can control your own heart rate.

Here's how to create the challenge:

Strength-building (weight-bearing) segments:

- Use light weights or no weights (body weight only) and lots of reps.
- Vary *eccentric* with *concentric* loading: Change up the pattern, tempo, and timing.
- Pulse-pulse-hold! This technique challenges the body. [*Disclaimer: isotonic exercise (holds and/or squeezes) can build up blood pressure. So do not do this if you have heart issues. And keep moving at all times so blood doesn't pool in your extremities.]

Cardio Segments:

The goal is SMART cardio movements (low-impact). Get your arms up over your head. This is a huge way to increase your heart rate!

(NOTE: Do not put arms over your head if you have heart problems. You can raise your arms, but to shoulder height, max. As always, run this program by your doctor first.)

For all Movements:

- Using the large muscles (like the leg muscles) while getting arms over head (keep arms at shoulder height max for cardiac patients) is a huge heart rate booster. So a combination of these movements (aka multi-joint movements) is a calorie-burner!
- Speed of movements can increase heart rate. For example, quick heel taps or toe taps.
- And of course, duration. Go as long as you can but don't overdo. Remember, we want you to feel as though you worked out—not be sore. I'd rather have you under-do than overdo.
- Intensity. You can do this in several ways. For example, simply add more effort. Or use a step, or employ greater range of motion. We can increase intensity without increasing impact!

This exercise program is so low-impact you can do it without shoes.

Summary: We are performing low-torque, low-impact movement that is effective and fun! And it challenges the mind and the body.

Everyone can do it!

Keys to Success and Sustainability

(Preventing Injury)

- **Form** is paramount! You MUST have proper form.
- **Stretch** in-between segments (optional).
- **Purposeful sequencing** of the segments.
- **Vary the tempo** of movements.
- **Reduce the torque**—lower weight and/or reduce lever (at first—you eventually *want* full range of motion).
- **Reduce the impact** (no jumping, no jarring).

Now we begin!

Regan MOVES Exercise Routine Synopsis

This full-body routine will change your life!

(Videos are on www.ReganMoves.com. You can subscribe to my online program there as well.)

Always check with your doctor before starting any exercise program. Stretches are optional. If you do stretch, keep it short and not too deep.

1. Warm Up and Stretch
2. Cardio: Soft Jacks and Stretch
3. Strength: Bicep Curls and Stretch
4. Cardio: Football Run and Stretch
5. Strength: Quads and Stretch
6. Cardio: Walk It Out, Heel Taps with Arms, and Stretch
7. Strength: Shoulders and Stretch
8. Cardio: Toe Taps and Stretch
9. Strength: Chest and Back and Stretch
10. Cardio: Taekwondo Punches and Stretch
11. Strength: Glutes and Hamstrings, Good Mornings, and Stretch
12. Abductors/Adductors
13. Strength/Cardio: The "Miley Cyrus" and Stretch
14. Cardio: Knee Lifts with Arms, Relax and Stretch
15. Strength: Calf Raises and Stretch (From a chair, one can also perform toe raises)

16. Cardio: The Skater and Stretch
17. Strength: Triceps and Stretch between each variation of the exercise

Now we move to the chair (if you are not seated already):

18. Strength: Lats and Stretch
19. Balance
20. Abdominals and Stretch
21. Full Body Stretch.

It is important to finish with a total body stretch, including the toes. It is important to again rotate your joints within the sockets (shoulders and hips) and to give full range of motion exercises for the joints.

I want you to take away a feeling of peace and relaxation as well as a strong sense of accomplishment for how you have worked out!

Regan MOVES Exercise Routine

With Detailed Descriptions and Modifications

(Videos are on www.ReganMoves.com. You can subscribe to my online program there as well.)

Let's get specific:

1. WARM UP: Dynamic Warm Up & ROM

Get your body moving for 3-5 minutes. Here we work the muscles that we will fully work during the workout. Perform a dynamic warmup. This means movement, not stretching (or do some light stretching at the end of the warmup). These can be bicep curls (with or without weights), walk on a spot, leg lifts, work the hamstrings, exercise the shoulders, and perform shoulder circles. Generally warm up your entire body.

Practice low-torque techniques the entire time. That is, do cardio and weight-bearing movements (without weights or with light weights) that mimic the movements you're going to do later (including the weight-lifting movements).

For example, you can do bicep curls without weights while walking on the spot. Or use one or two-pound weights. Warm up your legs, biceps, and shoulders. Do arm circles. Wrist circles. Hip circles and kicks. You can walk or jog on the spot. Warm up your whole body.

If your legs or knees are sore, you can warm up from a chair.

Modifications

Modify up: Use a step. Do not use risers for the step, though, as adding a step will slightly increase the torque on your knees (during each step-up and step-down). Risers will do so even more. Work up to this point and at your own pace.

Modify down: Perform from a chair.

Stretch. If comfortable, stretch your muscles after the dynamic warmup. Move the joints of the body (rotate joints in socket) from the neck to the fingers to the toes.

I briefly stretch my entire body, including my abs. I rotate the joints in my arms and hips. Don't forget to stretch your toes!

Note: To stretch quadriceps muscles from a chair, place foot under the chair and lean back.

2. SOFT JACKS

These are modified jumping jacks that are low-torque and low-impact. And you can perform them from a chair.

As you know, we don't perform any jumping (impactful) movements, and we don't add any torque throughout the workout.

Soft Jacks are simply walking on a spot or shallow squatting while moving your arms. They are a combination of leg work (walking on the spot) and arms. Walk on a spot and move your arms overhead.

In terms of range-of-motion (ROM), the arms can have a ROM comfortable for you. The legs can get interesting. If you're able to, I recommend you do a mini-squat (the degree to which you squat is entirely up to you and your ability) and add arms.

If you have knee issues or arthritis, you might want to remain in a fairly upright position. Or perform this exercise while seated: Stomp your feet and move your arms! This works great. Or alternate between toe taps and heel taps.

If you wish to squat in this movement: Again, we do not perform deep squats in this program—the torque on the knee is too high.

However, we can still present a challenge to, and further incorporate, the leg muscles by demonstrating safe, shallow squats which I call a mini-squat or pulse squat.

Here, because we will be leaning forward to reduce torque on the knee, it is important to protect the back. If you have back issues, do not squat and do not hinge too far forward.

For those who do not have back issues, here is your form when performing the mini-squat: Keep your back straight or slightly arched, not rounded. Draw your belly button to your spine.

Never hold your breath—always breathe. Try a sequence of squat-and-reach or step-step-reach movements and so on.

Modifications

Modify up: From a standing position, step and use arms or squat lower (as your knees allow) and use arms. Again, only squat slightly lower than the shallow pulse squat.

Modify down: To lower the intensity, perform from a chair. Step with the feet and use arms. Or simply do heel taps (or toe taps, or alternate heel taps with toe taps) with arms.

An alternative to toe taps or heel taps is simply toe raises (lift toes off the ground while your heels remain on the ground) or heel raises (vice versa) while you lift your arms.

Or move either the arms or the legs depending on your comfort level.

Stretch.

> **Spoiler Alert!**
> Just the smallest tweak to your form or how you hold your body can allow you to perform the exercise!
> **The Beauty is in the Details**

3. BICEP CURLS

Pretty standard. One thing to watch for is hyperextension of the elbow or wrist. People with chronic conditions tend to be susceptible to hyperextension of the joints. Their joints can be very vulnerable in this position so please be cognizant of this. Consider not completely straightening your arms, at least at first. Don't lock your elbow joints.

Tempo Trick: Get your muscles "thinking" by changing up the tempo on both concentric and eccentric loading. Strength increases much more quickly when we incorporate eccentric loading.

For example, I will do beats of 4: 4 slow, then 3-2-1-UP, then 3-2-1 DOWN then 2 and 2.

This ties into:

> **Work smarter, not harder!**

Second Trick: Do a small set then stretch. Then repeat a set. In between sets reevaluate your weights and go heavier or lighter. That way you get more work done.

Third Trick: Pulse and hold!

> **Important**
> The day after your workout you want to feel like "you worked out," not be sore. So don't overdo it!

Modifications

Modify up: Increase the weight, ROM, or number of reps (duration). I do this still, and it's how I got started.

Modify down: Use a lower range of motion (don't extend your arms so much), don't use weights, or lighten the weights (use tuna cans or soup cans). Make sure you hold your hand such that the angle of your wrist and hand remains neutral. It should be comfortable. You are the boss. Be responsible (you choose your position).

Stretch the biceps. There are a few ways you can do this standing or from a chair: from the floor (seated, with arms behind you mostly straight and lean back) or using a wall. You can also extend arms out and pull fingers down with palms up.

4. FOOTBALL RUN

Take two wide steps laterally away from the body and then take two narrow steps in (out-out-in-in/wide-wide-narrow-narrow). Remember, don't step too far outside the frame of the body. We want to keep the torque low on the knees.

Modifications

Modify up: Go faster!

Modify down: Perform from a chair. Tap your feet or step. Take gentle steps to the side in the same format, out-out-in-in.

You could also do heel raises and toe raises repeatedly or in an alternating fashion. It's a brain teaser. And it's fun!

Tip: Use music! You can do it to the beat of your favorite song. Do beats of 4 in an out-out-in-in step sequence.

Stretch (optional). Stretch the quads, as before. You can stretch from a standing position where you grab your foot (or pant leg) which makes it easier. Or do a swimmer's stretch: One foot in front, one behind, and gently lean back. Stretch the hips and glutes.

5. PULSE SQUATS (my favorite!)

This is a calorie burner! That's because it uses the large muscles. Remember the form we use for the squat? Use it here! In this exercise we do gentle, shallow squats in a repetitive manner to get the heart rate up and the legs working.

Here's where we modify a traditional lunge. You can isolate a leg simply by transferring weight to it. To achieve this you can (almost imperceptibly) shift your weight to the other leg. Even just a small shift in weight can increase intensity to that leg!

To do this, go up on one toe (on the opposite leg). Or if you're feeling strong, you can even lift that foot off the ground!

> **The Beauty is in the Details**
> Even just a small shift in weight can isolate one leg, allowing you to perform the exercise and get results.

Modifications

Modify up: Go deeper and/or add weights. Use a greater range of motion, and/or keep time under tension (don't stand all the way up between pulses). Be aware of your body. Don't overdo.

Modify down: You can do shallower squats. Or just transfer your weight. Simply standing and transferring weight from one leg to the other is a very effective way to build strength. When the knees are sore and this is all you can do, that's OK! You're doing it!

You're doing things that keep you active. When you are ready, perform this exercise at a greater range of motion.

> **My Knee Surgeon's Advice**
> Perform bent-leg lifts, knee extensions, and hip flexions from a chair. Use changes in tempo to make it challenging. You can add weights.

He said, "If you don't start doing these exercises, you're going to need a double knee replacement in 10 years."

Guess what? I took his advice—and I didn't need knee surgery!

> **TIP:** Your bathtub makes it fun and easy—use the buoyancy of the water to perform these exercises!

(SLOW)   and   (LOW)

Slow tempo increases tension and decreases risk of injury

Low range of motion decreases torque and risk of injury

Intensity for any of these exercises can be changed with tempo, pattern, weight, and range of motion. To lower intensity, use a chair. To raise it, add a step if appropriate. (No risers)

Refresher

Two tricks to raising your heart rate—pulse and tempo:

- Pulse-and-hold can be performed with any cardio or strength exercise.
- You can also use time-under-tension as a way to increase your heart rate.

Note: You can perform Pulse Squats with no weights. Keep your feet closer together to reduce torque on knees.

To modify up, add weights!

Important and very effective: To modify down, perform leg lifts from a chair. Do the knee surgeon's exercises! Just be careful not to lock your knees when doing knee extensions.

Stretch (optional). I always stretch after leg exercises.

6. WALK-IT-OUT

A frequently-used cardio segment, Walk-it-Out is simply that—simply walk on a spot (with knees as high as you would like to lift) to get that heart rate up in a safe fashion. Arms can be used above or to the side to get the heart rate up even more.

Add punches if you like, or any other fun sequence of arm movements. Alternate with Heel Taps with Arms if you like.

Modifications

Modify up: Add a step and/or weights.

Modify down: Perform from a chair to take it down a notch.

7. SHOULDERS

Some of my favorite exercises. We exercise the shoulder in all planes to target all of the areas of the shoulder. Shoulder press, mini-raises, rotate about the joint.

Be very mindful of rotator cuff issues and be ready to modify. Reduce the lever if needed. This can be done in all planes.

Overhead Press

I usually start with an overhead press. And remember the tip of pulse-pulse-hold? As well as tempo variations? I incorporate these in every workout. It keeps it fun, safe, and effective.

For the shoulder press say to yourself (where pulse is at shoulder height), "pulse-pulse-press," "pulse-pulse-pulse-press," and so on. And you can do it in reverse ("press-press-down"). And you can do "pulse-pulse-pulse-hold" (or "press-press-hold") where you hold at the top of the movement.

I perform pulse-press and pulse-hold sequences not only at full range of motion (for those who can do it), but also at the top-of-the-head height (arms not fully extended upward). This increases time under tension, and is a great strength-building exercise if you're able to do it. Stretch.

Modification

Modify down: Reduce or eliminate weights. Take rests, start slow, or do one arm at a time. If it hurts, stop.

Shoulder Raises

Raise to the side and front. Stretch.

Modification (this one is excellent!)

Bend the arm and simply pivot (rotate) the weight (free weight or body weight, which is just your arm) about the shoulder. Palms may face the body or face away from the body.

This is one of the best exercises for people with shoulder pain or impingement.

Lateral Deltoid

Extend arms to the side or at a 45-degree angle for comfort. Perform raises, including mini-raises near the top (shoulder height), and perform pulse and hold. Stretch.

Modification

Bend the arms! Feel the difference?

Stretch. Palms against or towards wall, and lean away from wall.

Again, feel free to bend your arms. This decreases torque and increases comfort. Now, in performing the exercise you'll look like you're doing "chicken wings"! This can actually be another source of levity during your workout.

Remember, the beauty's in the details, and these small changes translate to BIG results. The goal is to get the muscle working in whatever comfortable way you can.

Posterior Deltoid (the back of the shoulder)

Here you may be able to perform reverse flys. Do so to your comfort level. Stretch.

Modification

Again, feel free to decrease the lever by increasing the bend of the elbow, such that the forearms are nearly touching the arms. If this causes discomfort in the elbow, find a happy medium. Another modification—don't bring your arms up so high.

> All these exercises can (and should) be repeated in sets. And you can stretch between sets. This is how we are able to *build muscle*. We use high reps and low (or no) weights.

One of my mottos is:

> **Slow and Low**
> Slow tempo and low range-of-motion
> *Slow and Steady Wins the Race!*

Following these principles allows more reps!

That's why Regan MOVES is effective.

To stretch the shoulders, use the wall as a "buddy." There are four ways to modify the stretch:

- Change hand height
- Change angle at which you turn from the wall
- Change the body's nearness to the wall
- Change hand position (palm facing towards or away from the wall)

As you change your hand position, palms to the wall will increase the stretch in the bicep. The back of the hand to the wall will increase the shoulder stretch. Fist to the wall will give you a little bit of both.

Tip: One can perform these stretches overhead. Simply raise one arm (and lean to opposite side if desired to increase the stretch) and rotate the arm in the socket for a real "feel good" stretch of that shoulder and bicep.

Stretch/Rotate: Rotate the shoulder in the joint with your hand above you or below. It feels good.

8. TOE TAPS

You can perform these from a standing position or from a chair. If you're reticent or have pain, you may simply raise your heels while toes remain on the floor.

Do them at half time or double speed to change your tempo/intensity.

Stretch your toes: Rock left and right from big toe to little toe. The higher you lift your heel off the ground the further back your toes will bend so be careful with this stretch.

Modifications

Modify up: Increase tempo, add weights, or add bounce (not jumps) if knees/hips allow. Stretch. Bouncing is OK. It builds bones.

Modify down: As in the standing position, if you do this exercise from the chair, you can either tap the toe or heel while the foot is off the floor, or simply raise the heels/toes in alternating fashion. I highly recommend a chair if your knees are sore.

9. CHEST AND BACK

Chest: Wall or Barre Pushups

Wall Pushups are one of my favorites! Here, form is very important. The angle at which your wrists are engaged with the wall is important.

Wall pushups are an excellent way to do a pushup because you don't have to get on the floor and you still get a great workout! In fact, they're much easier (less torque) on the shoulders so I call them a smart way to do a pushup.

Here's the thing about pushups. Even if you do knee-pushups, pushups put a lot of torque on the shoulder joint as you can imagine. For wall pushups, the further the feet are from the wall the more intensity you will feel.

Be mindful of your form. Your back should be straight, your body should be straight (as possible), neck and head in line with the body.

Modifications

Vary the tempo. Focus on eccentric and concentric loading. You can even do explosive pushups where you push as hard and fast as you can away from the wall.

Stretch. Use the wall to stretch. Palms pressing the wall stretches the biceps. Back of hand or fist pressing the wall stretches the shoulder. Play with the angle you stand to the wall and the height at which you hold your arm/place hand. You can also do arm circles for a feel-good stretch.

For less torque and less intensity, simply stand closer to the wall. It still counts!

Everything you DO counts!

You can also use a barre (or table, desk, or other surface) for pushups. Make it the right height for you. The same techniques apply. The further your feet are from the barre (or table, etc.), the more intensity you will feel, the more torque on the shoulders. Again, keep your neck and body straight, your head in line with your body.

Chest Press

While standing or seated, hold a weight close to your chest with both hands. Extend it forward at shoulder height and bring it back in.

Back: Rows

From a standing position, hold your arms at a 45-degree angle or where it's comfortable. Perform the rows. From a seated position you can hinge at the hip if possible (all the while protecting your back by drawing your belly button into your spine as you keep your back fairly straight).

Draw weights (or arms) back. Squeeze the shoulder blades together at the top of the movement. For comfort you can perform one arm at a time. In terms of finding the right position or range of motion, your comfort is number one.

To increase intensity hinge more at the hips (lean further forward), lifting your weights in a more vertical line. Stretch.

You can squeeze at the top and/or you can hold. You can even pulse and hold. Remember, squeezing can raise blood pressure so take care and use caution.

Modification for Chest

I love this modification, and I love the name—the bear hug! From a standing or seated position, hold your arms in front of you, preferably at shoulder height (if comfortable). Then draw them out to the side, stretching the chest as it's comfortable. Bring arms back center and then down. This can be performed with or without weights.

Further Modification: I've had clients (one in particular who had a frozen shoulder) keep arms at their sides then bend the elbow and still be able to stretch out the chest and ribcage from that position, slowly bringing the arms back to center.

It's still a very effective exercise!

DO what you can WHEN you can!

Another Modification for Chest is wall pushups where you stand closer to the wall.

To modify up, use a barre, bench, or a barbell in the rack, or even the floor. If you opt for the floor, you can do the pushups from knees or toes.

Elbows out can put more torque on the shoulder. You should have an elbow position according to your comfort level.

I don't recommend doing pushups using a fist. It puts too much torque on the wrist. But bottom line, do what works best for you, including hand position.

Stretch: Use the wall to stretch. Put your hand against the wall and with a straight arm, turn away from the wall. Palm against the wall will stretch the biceps. The back of the hand (or fist) against the wall will stretch your shoulder.

Experiment with the angle you stand in relation to the wall. Experiment also with the height you place your hand. You can do arm circles to loosen up as well. Repeat another set. Stretch.

10. TAEKWONDO PUNCHES

Super fun—simply squat and punch! As long as the squat is performed with proper form you can add a squat to the punches. These are fun! Punch fast!

Be careful not to injure the elbow by punching too fast, or hyperextending the joint by extending your arm too far out.

Modifications

Modify up: Add light weights. Just be careful with the twist of your wrist at the end of the punch.

Modify down: Take away the squat and just stand and punch. Breathe out with the punches. Perform from a chair. From the chair, just punch. Or stomp and punch, or knee lift and punch! Fun! Stretch.

11. GLUTES AND HAMSTRINGS

Let's do Good Mornings. These are a great exercise if they're within your ability. Stand and hinge at the hip. (Be sure to draw your belly button to the spine to protect your back). Simply lean forward.

Your back should be flat or slightly arched, not rounded. Lean forward.

You can support yourself by placing a hand on your leg—in fact, this is recommended. Slowly bring the trunk back up to standing position. If you have back issues, modify and/or do from a chair (you have more control over your ROM and can place weight on your hands).

Modifications

Modify down: Stand behind a chair and use it for balance. Extend one leg behind you and bring back to neutral. You can even pulse-and-hold, or extend-then-release then bring back to neutral.

You can also start with a bend in the knee and extend (straighten) the leg towards the wall. Add flexion to the foot to increase intensity. Stretch.

Here's a great glute exercise for those with back issues: While seated, squeeze glutes. Squeeze three or four times, take a break then squeeze again. Squeeze and hold. Stretch.

Be careful not to do too many of these. Isometric exercises can cause blood to pool in the extremities.

Exciting modification—Gentle hamstrings: This is great for seniors and those with limited mobility. From a seated position, step out with foot in front and draw it back to starting position. Or draw it under your chair. Or lift knee slightly (standing or seated) and draw heel to glute. Stretch.

12. ABDUCTORS/ADDUCTORS

This point in the routine is a good time to perform mobility of the hip, working the outside (abductors) and inside (adductors) muscles of the legs. These are from a standing position.

Abductors (outer leg muscles): Perform gentle lateral leg raises to the side, then stretch.

Adductors (inner thigh muscles): Cross the body with the leg. Stretch. I suggest you alternate legs after each movement to avoid fatigue.

Modifications

Abductors: While seated, simply step out to the side then back to center.

Adductors: While seated, cross your leg over your other knee or ankle.

Important: This is a good place to stretch the hips. I call it the Special Stretch. It moves the stretch from the inner thigh, to the hamstrings, to the outer thigh, hip, and glute, to the back. (See the photos on page 60.) It feels so good!

If the knee feels sore in any of these stretches or the tendon feels taut, I recommend flexing the foot (bring toes up) to release tension in the knee tendon (if this does not create discomfort for the calf).

13. STRENGTH/CARDIO MIX

This is a fun one! I call it the *Miley Cyrus* because I like performing it to the beat of her song "Party in the USA"!

Start by doing heel taps with arms in front of you at shoulder height (bend and/or lower your arm if you have shoulder problems or want to reduce the torque). Do four beats of each: palms down, palms together, palms up, palms together. It's a brain-teaser!

Remember, you can incorporate lots of cross-movements: opposite arm to opposite leg, then same arm to same leg. It gets you thinking and having fun!

This is an example of how your comfort can be increased while still having fun exercising in this challenging move. With arms in front at shoulder height (or lower if that is more comfortable), the arms can be straight or bent. You can alternate with heel taps. For fun, change up the pattern of palms up, palms down, palms together. Stretch.

14. KNEE LIFTS WITH ARMS

Again, have fun with this pattern! A familiar dance-type step I like to use is 1-2-3-LIFT! (step-step-step-knee lift). If your hip flexors are tight or your quads are sore, just make the knee lift a step (or toe tap or heel tap). Perform at your own tempo.

Modifications

Don't lift the knees too high.

Perform from a chair. Use heel raises and toe taps instead of knee lifts.

15. CALF RAISES

For those with gastrocnemius, soleus or Achilles tendon issues, make sure to get approval before trying this exercise. Start slowly with a low range of motion. Also, if you have sore knees, I recommend not doing this from a standing position. Instead, follow the modifications.

Stand on your tippy-toes. Hold. To isolate each leg, instead of going onto your tippy-toes right off the bat for just one leg, I recommend going to both tippy toes first (raising both heels to get on your toes), then lifting one foot off the floor and lowering the opposite leg. It just seems to be easier on the toes.

To ease the intensity of this exercise, use the chair or wall more extensively and simply slightly transfer weight from one leg to the other while going up on your toes.

Modifications

From a chair, raise your heel off the floor to a height comfortable for you. Alternate feet. Be sure to stretch. You can alternately raise the heel then lift the toes to stretch.

Going to one's toes while seated is a fine modification of this exercise. And if your toes are injured and can't sustain a lot of weight, this modification is recommended.

If you have sore knees, rock back on your heels then forward with your weight slightly shifted towards your toes. You can do this from a chair for further modification.

Stretch, including the toes! Spread toes on floor, and roll back and forth from pinky toe to big. You might want to do it with your shoes off.

16. THE SKATER

You'll look like a speed-skater! Extend each leg alternately to the side while swinging the arms in the opposite direction. If safe for your back, you may slightly hinge at the hip.

This is a fun exercise that gets the heart rate up and creates a challenge. To maintain safety of the knees, keep your weight over the knee of the planted leg.

Modification

Do a lower range of motion—don't step out to the side as far—or perform from a chair. Stretch.

17. TRICEPS

With this exercise I am careful not to over-stress the shoulder, so I start with kickbacks. Hinge at the hip for a more intense exercise or, if your shoulders or back are sore, simply carry out the exercise from a more upright position. We are still working the muscle.

If you have chronic fatigue syndrome or fibromyalgia, a common issue is a sore upper back and neck muscles. When performing these and other exercises, be sure to relax the neck.

Also, make sure to include neck stretches. These are particularly useful during exercises such as reverse flys, triceps exercises, and exercises for the back.

(See the photos on p. 62-63 for great neck stretches.)

Pulse and Hold

This is gonna get them burning!

Triceps may continue with swimmers and overhead extensions.

Modifications

Modify up: Use heavier weights.

Modify down: Decrease weights. Complete the exercise(s) from a chair while leaning forward as much as you want. Stay upright and/or lower your ROM. Or do isometric holds.

For kick-backs and swimmers: Pulse and hold or just squeeze.

Overhead extensions: Stretch between each variation of the exercise.

18. LATS

If you have shoulder, neck, or back issues, I encourage stretching instead—still do the exercise but without weights. Just feel the stretch.

While seated, extend both arms overhead (let's call this center or neutral position). You may hold a weight if you like. What I do is hold one dumbbell between both hands, with the bells in each hand.

From neutral, lean back ever so gently (if comfortable and safe for your back). Move your arms behind your head ever so gently (if this movement is OK for you) as much as is comfortable. Come back to center/neutral above the head.

Next, move the arms back and slightly to one side.

Let's start with the left side. When moving your arms left, go until your right arm grazes your right ear. From that position, slightly take the arms behind your head, then return them to the plane of your head. You should feel a stretch along your right side.

Move the arms back to neutral position (directly above your head).

Now go to the other side. Move the arms right until your left arm grazes your left ear. From that position, slightly take the arms back and then back up on that same angle. You'll feel a stretch along your left side. Move the arms back to neutral. Stretch. Remember, this can be performed with or without weights.

People find this to be a very relaxing exercise. It is an enjoyable movement. So if it is reasonable, safe, and comfortable for you, I encourage you to try it. Stretch.

19. BALANCE

While seated or standing, hold your arms out to the side or in front of you. Look to your left, look to your right. Increase the challenge by closing your eyes. Or just close your eyes and don't look left or right. Breathe in through the nose and out through the mouth.

Next, do this exercise combination while lifting one foot up off the floor.

Another variation: While standing, hold arms out to the side or in front of you, go up on your toes. Look to your left, look to your right.

Try closing your eyes.

For a challenge, try this (eyes open and closed) with just one foot on the ground and on toes!

A further challenge is to have the feet displaced front to back in a walking stance. I challenge you to stay steady on this one!

Modification

From a chair with arms out to the side, look to your left and then right. Add a twist at the waist.

Lean! This is so good for your obliques and for balance. From a chair, lean gently to your side and see how you feel. Try it with eyes open and closed. It is important to keep your back straight and your head, hips, and knees square. Avoid twisting or bending the spine. Take a few deep breaths in through the nose and out through the mouth.

20. ABDOMINALS

This is probably my favorite part of the program. This is a wonderful and effective way to build and maintain the muscles of your entire core! Including the *rectus abdominis* (abs) and trunk. And they can all be done from a chair!

From a chair, we start with a plank. Hold the legs out (do not lock your knees.) Then we add kicks in three different ways:

1. Butterfly kicks up and down
2. Legs cross over each other at the knee or ankle
3. Legs out and in laterally

Then it might be time for some slow sit-ups—slow on the way up and on the way down. Remember to breathe in through the nose and out through the mouth.

Next we perform gentle twists. Hold arms to the side in a 180-degree fashion. Drop arms if shoulders are sore, and turn slightly and gently. Breathe out through the mouth as you gently turn, breathe in through the nose as you come back to center. This is a relaxing exercise and is very good for the waist.

Move on to obliques, the Lean-and-Hold. This is one of my favorite exercises. Head, shoulders, hips, knees, and feet should be square. Don't bend or twist your spine. Just lean to the side and hold. Be sure to breathe. Lean both ways a couple of times. It is OK to leave your feet on the floor for this, although a lot of people lift them off the ground.

Big circles are another fan favorite. These target the entire trunk. Lean forward and do a circle all the way around. (You may want to support your back by placing your hands on your knees while leaning forward.) Take good care if you have back issues.

Little circles are next. Same thing, just with a smaller ROM.

Stretch the back. Place a *C-curve* in your spine. Drop your chin to your chest while curving your spine. Exhale through the mouth. Roll back up. If on a mat, you may do a little-piece-of-heaven (cat) stretch.

Take a deep breath in through the nose, blow out through the mouth.

(For more stretching, please participate in my online exercise class! Find the details on www.ReganMoves. com.)

We are now approaching the final steps of the exercise program, the relaxing phase. In the final minutes of our class, prepare for a gentle balancing segment.

Kick out ABS—simply balance. Don't put weight on your shoulders and elbows.

Tip: I recommend you have some core, leg and quad strength to help carry out the exercises as I have laid them out. You can achieve this very successfully with Pilates. Many moves in Pilates incorporate both the quad muscles and the abdominal muscles simultaneously:

- The V—with one leg or both. If too difficult, bend your knees.
- Lower Abs—Lay on the floor on your back. Lift both legs up to 90-degrees, and back down. Bend the knees to make it easier. If performing from a chair, lift legs (either bent or straight) to hip height. Can lift one or both legs at once.

Way to go! You did it! You just completed a pretty extensive workout!

Let's take some time to celebrate, calm your mind, and set yourself up for success for the rest of the day.

> **Think about what you are grateful for as you breathe in each time!**

Take three deep breaths of gratitude.

Breathe air in deeply, stretch arms overhead, and let it out as you drop your arms.

21. STRETCHING

Finish with total body stretching—including the toes—and deep breathing.

It is important to again rotate the joints within the sockets (shoulders and hips) and to give full range of motion exercises for the joints. We want you feel peace, relaxation, and a strong sense of accomplishment for how you have just worked out!

Swimmer's Stretch

This one is very beneficial for stretching the quads and calves. Feel the stretch in the back leg. Increase comfort by lifting heel off the ground. Change the stretch by tucking in the seat.

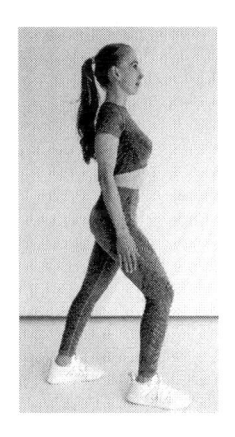

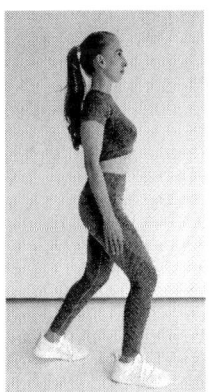

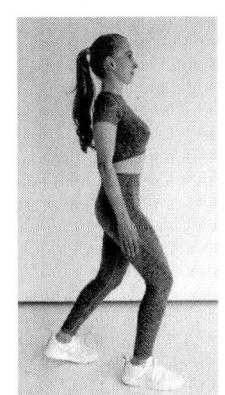

"Special" Stretch for hips and hamstrings

This is my own Special Stretch. Perform from a seated position. It really stretches the back, the hip flexors, and buttocks.

The stretch begins with the back of leg and moves towards the hip. Lower the head, as in the last picture and/or lean forward (in every stage) to augment the stretch. Sit up when moving the leg. Put your hands on your knees when leaning forward to support your back.

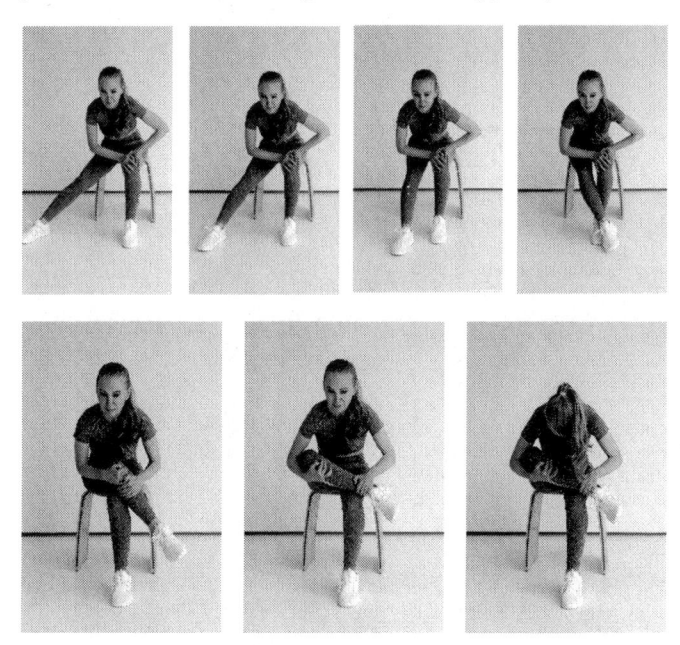

If you like, you can do this stretch on the mat—it will really stretch the hip flexor. So you're getting all sides of the hip in that stretch.

Sit down when stretching abductors. It puts less pressure on the knees.

Abs and Back Stretch

From a chair, lean back and stretch. If your back allows, you may arch it—and you may add arms overhead. Or just put arms overhead and don't arch the back. Breathe in through the nose, out through the mouth. Feel that air all the way down to the bottom of your tummy.

(I have to do an exaggerated abs stretch and really arch my back. This is because my back is naturally overly-arched. So I must increase the ROM that much more to stretch my abs.)

For the piece-of-heaven stretch (if on floor) you may not want to take your butt all the way back to your heels. Just stay in the position where your back feels "stretchiest."

Shoulder Stretch

For the backs of shoulders, reach arms up on a wall and lean away from it. For the front of your shoulders, pull one arm across your body. Another option for front and back is to find something the right height (I use my ottoman and sit down on the floor and lower my body) to feel the stretch.

Don't forget to rotate your wrists and neck as well.

Rotate arms in socket with arms over head (see next page):

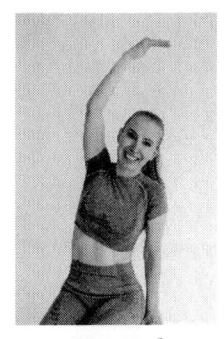

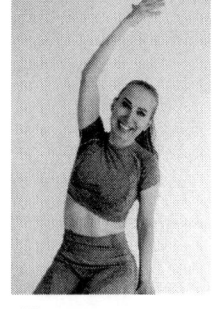

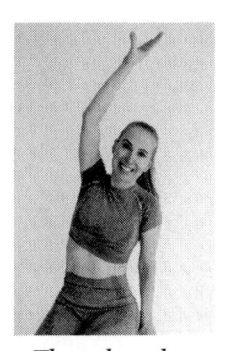

Neutral   *Rotate one way*   *Then the other*

You can also do this stretch with arms at your side instead of overhead.

I like stretching my neck last—it is the most relaxing of the stretches.

My three favorite neck stretches are what I call the Look, Lean and Robot:

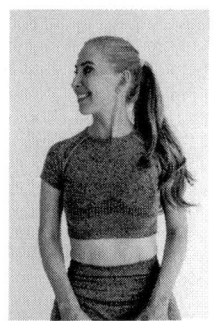

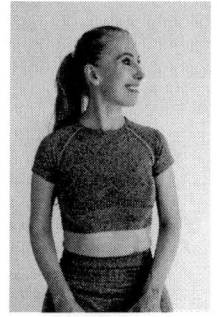

Look *to your right and hold, look to your left and hold*

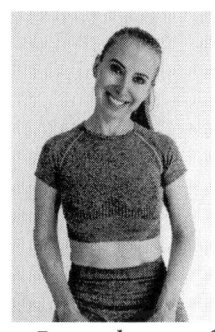

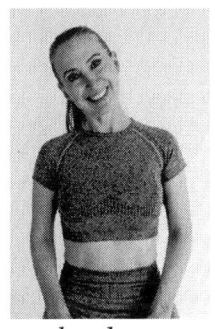

Lean *the top of your head to one shoulder and hold, then the other*

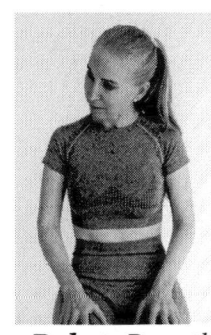

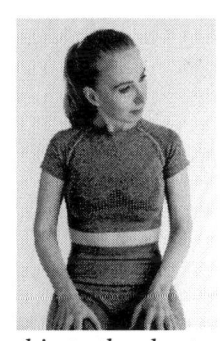

Robot: *Drop the chin to the chest, then rotate the chin to one shoulder. Repeat on the other side. It's like a robot pivoting its head on its axis. You can even make the "err, err" sound!*

If approved by your doctor, you can augment the Look stretch by pushing your head further with your hand.

Nice job stretching!

Recap

Form: The main goal is to maintain a low-torque position. This will help keep you safe. It will prevent injury and you'll be able to do the exercises without exacerbating your pain. Eventually your pain will go down and your strength and energy will go up.

Regan MOVES helps you exercise the muscles that support the joints. As your strength increases, you'll gain stability and longevity of the joints and increase overall quality of life. Studies show that the longterm effects of moderate exercise include decreased inflammation, which decreases your pain.

Regan MOVES helps people increase energy and decrease pain.

Eliminate fatigue by stretching frequently if it helps.

Keeping the segments short (1-3 minutes tops) helps prevent fatigue.

Changing up the exercises frequently helps you maintain energy so you can carry out the entire sequence of exercises.

Keeping the extremities within the frame of the body helps reduce torque.

Great job! ENJOY the fruits of your labor!

Regan MOVES Levels

Regan MOVES is available in three different levels—Gentle, Intermediate, and Advanced. Remember, we want you to start slow and work your way up when you feel ready.

> Join me online and let's exercise together:
> *www.ReganMoves.com*

Regan MOVES Gentle

Regan MOVES Gentle is for those just starting out or those who experience extreme fatigue, pain, and/or disease activity.

All are low-intensity exercises done from a chair. You'll feel better by doing the moves and will gain strength. You can modify up to the different levels as you feel ready.

Regan MOVES Intermediate

Regan MOVES Intermediate provides a moderate level of intensity. It is still low-torque and low-impact yet very effective. Some exercises are performed from a chair.

Most lupus and arthritis patients who are in some degree of remission or have some ability for movement fall into this category. They work their way up to Regan MOVES Advanced.

Regan MOVES Advanced

This is the highest level of intensity. Still low-torque and low-impact, this exciting level is safe for the joints.

We show you how to intensify your workout while still remaining safe. We do this in several ways including using a step, increasing range of motion (ROM), adding more weights, or all of the above. It is the quickest way to burn calories and lose weight!

Note: It is important to keep joint safety as your highest priority. Therefore do not get ahead of yourself. Stay at a level that keeps you comfortable. You should not have pain. Each person will monitor themselves. Trust yourself. That's why minimizing torque is so important.

You can always increase ROM so start slow. The gist of Regan MOVES is to learn how to minimize torque and implement these techniques during exercise and daily life—from standing close to a shelf before removing an item to properly opening a jar.

The goal is for your exercise to be repeatable.

Repeatable = Success

That's why EASY is Effective!

Regan's Story

Regan Birr is a mechanical engineer who began her career as a patent agent. She is a certified personal trainer, group fitness instructor and coach.

Regan is the founder and executive director of the Lupus Research Foundation (LRF) in Minnesota. She has served on the board of the Lupus Foundation of Colorado and worked with the Lupus Foundation of Northern California.

She lives with her husband Todd near Minneapolis, Minnesota. She is a musician, national anthem soloist, and motivational speaker. With Todd, Regan competes at the national level in the Olympic ice sport of curling.

She is a healthy lupus patient—in remission on medication, living well. Regan enjoys advocating for lupus awareness.

The LRF is the home of *Lupus Spiel USA*, a pro-am curling tournament that is the largest of its kind in the world. It raises funds for lupus research and awareness.

Regan was diagnosed with *systemic lupus erythematosus* causing *WHO Class IV diffuse proliferative glomerulonephritis*—kidney lupus. She was technically put into remission after starting her treatment. But she had to stay on her treatment to achieve long-lasting remission.

Her treatment consisted of a two-and-a-half year regimen of cyclophosphamide (Cytoxan), a breast cancer chemotherapy. Cytoxan was used to reduce the overactive nature of her immune system.

During this time she continued to struggle with clinical symptoms including severe pain, fatigue, and (looking back) depression. Her joint pain sometimes precluded her from walking even short distances and she had no stamina. She needed a cane to get up the stairs. Her fatigue level was such that walking was a challenge—she had to stop and take a break after taking only a few steps. Holding conversations was difficult. She struggled with weight gain due to prednisone and inactivity.

After getting fed up having to use a cane to climb the stairs, Regan decided she had to make a change. She changed her diet which got her energy levels up again. Then she really ramped up her life and got rid of her pain once she started exercising. Now she enjoys a life of freedom and happiness.

Please share this story with others, and share your story! You will inspire people around you and motivate them to lead better lives. Together we will all lead better lives—lives we were meant to live that we've created for ourselves.

REGAN MOVES™

Summary

Regan MOVES emphasizes joint safety and exercises that are doable and won't exacerbate pain. It also accommodates those dealing with fatigue.

That is why the order and nature of the segments is so important. It can help a person sustain exercise at their own pace without fatiguing them further. It can actually help them create energy.

Regan MOVES helps people increase energy and decrease pain.

In addition to the movement helping people increase their energy, long-term effects of moderate exercise include reducing inflammation.

The exercises can be as intense as you want them to be.

The theory behind Regan MOVES and the teachings about torque make exercise functional, from opening a jar to going up and down the stairs.

The program is applicable to those with recent joint injuries and surgeries. Regan has worked with people with fused vertebrae, frozen shoulders, and pain.

A frequent comment we hear from people is they don't

feel like they were working "that hard." That they felt that they worked out but weren't sore. And they'd look at their watch and see they had burned a bunch of calories while the time flew!

These are things we want for you. These are the goals of Regan MOVES:

- For you to feel like you worked out, but not be sore.
- And for you to feel energized!

For more information go to:
www.ReganMOVES.com
www.ReganBirr.com
www.LetsCureLupus.org

Books coming soon:

Regan MOVES: The Little Manual of Effective Eating

Regan MOVES: The Little Manual of Healthy Mindset

Easy is Effective: You Have the Power to Feel Better and Change Your Life by Following a Few Simple Step

REGAN MOVES™

Services

In addition to online exercise programs, Regan also offers services as a motivational coach. Following the recommendations of the client's physician and other healthcare providers, Regan helps implement these plans for wellness.

Regan is a keynote speaker. Her topics include:

- "Shine Your Light: For You, and For Others" is a motivational speech about overcoming adversity and the power of the human spirit.
- "EASY is Effective, Move to Better-Than-Ever" is a talk that outlines why repeatability leads to success. It provides simple tools to help give us those daily wins.
- "Teamwork: Lessons On Ice" talks about how the best teammates we know are those who know themselves, and have the desire and care to learn how to listen to their teammates for optimal teamwork and success.

The keynote topics can be tailored to your specific needs and audience.

Regan conducts workshops. Typically these include a demonstration of her exercise program, a talk, and a segment on nutrition and mental health. They too can be tailored to your needs and schedule.

If you would be open to a conversation about a Regan MOVES keynote speech, workshop, or both, please reach out to Regan.

A portion of the proceeds from Regan MOVES services goes to the Lupus Research Foundation, a charitable organization whose mission is to help cure lupus by raising awareness and funds for research.

Endorsements

"Regan MOVES is very valuable for people who need safe movements to help them build strength and endurance and reduce pain. I recommend this program to my patients who need low impact, effective movements to accomplish their goals. I love the movements and the education that is provided on torque and biomechanics. This is beneficial for individuals with different chronic conditions, comorbidities or other factors that would complicate their ability to move."

~ *David Anderson, Doctor of Physical Therapy*

"I know about the struggles people have with lupus; it is near and dear to my heart. Regan's book will help people get fit even if they didn't think they could. Her approach fosters community and like-mindedness, and since she's walked the walk, she relates to people in a way few coaches can. The program is thorough and unique. I know what it takes to be a good coach and the importance of great communication for your team. Regan provides that to her MOVERS."

~ *Pam Borton, MCC, NBC-HWC, Executive High Performance Coach, Final Four Basketball Coach, Winningest Basketball Coach at the University of Minnesota, Two-Time Nominee Naismith Coach of the Year, Certified Global Team Coach, Professional Speaker, Two-Time Author, Board of Trustees*

"Having a great interest in biomechanics and exercise/rehab, I can say that Regan's program is mechanically sound and can help people with mobility issues get moving. It's also a great way to start exercising again after injury or surgery. It can even act as a lighter workout between heavier workouts, and is a cardio/strength full-body, comprehensive workout."

~ *Dr. Greg DeNunzio, B.S. Engineering, M.S. Kinesiology and Exercise Science, M.S. Functional and Integrative Nutrition, Doctorate of Chiropractic, Owner of Marco Chiropractic Clinic/Optimize Health 360*

"Regan's book provides an excellent structure to maintain a healthy lifestyle with an easy and effective program."

~ *Eve Muirhead OBE, Olympic Champion, World Champion, Team GB Chef De Mission Milano Cortina 2026*

"Regan's intention is clear. She wants to bring relief, and inspiration, to those suffering with lupus, fibromyalgia, and depression. The program outlined in this book is a major contribution to a silent epidemic—and definitely MOVES me."

~ *Judy Katz, award-winning ghostwriter, book publisher and promoter*

"I am happy to endorse this program because I feel it will help many of my patients with rheumatological conditions and general pain and fatigue. Having been Regan's physician, I have seen her care and conscientiousness towards other people."

~ *Amy Elliott, MD Rheumatology and Internal Medicine, member of the American College of Physicians, Fellow of the American College of Rheumatology*

"I love the book and techniques in it. I believe it will be useful. Lupus "hits" close to home and this program provides space for people with challenges to still work out and retain their competitive spirit. It is a thoughtful and thorough program and I recommend it."

~Michael Roos, NFL All-Pro Offensive Tackle

Client Testimonials

"Your workouts are The Best because of the make-up of the routine, but also because you are dazzling and kind!" ~ *Andrea*

"I want to thank you so much for coming to the Lupus Foundation last week and showing us some easy exercises. I have not been sore from doing the exercises and I have lost a pound and a half in the past week. Like I said at the end of the class, it is very encouraging! Keep up the good work!" ~ *Joyce*

"Regan MOVES has helped me more in the past two years than anything I've tried in the past 6 years! I have lost 50 pounds and found things I actually like eating. Her coaching and encouragement have kept me going...I've even been able to do some house cleaning without pain! The Tuesday/Thursday MOVES class is not very long, but it's a fantastic workout. I started doing this completely in a chair, now I can do parts of it standing. Regan MOVES, you're a God-send in my life. THANK YOU!!" ~ *Valerie*

"I want to thank you for offering to do your class. You are the best instructor and so caring. Thank you for the good workout. I felt so much better when I left your class. You're a godsend! I really appreciate you and your fitness program." ~ *Carmen*

"At the age of 71 I was diagnosed with lupus. As soon as my medications took effect my doctor told me to look into some exercise to help counter some of the symptoms of the disease. Right after that the swim and tennis club to which I belong advertised a new class, given by Regan, for those with diseases like lupus, MS, and chronic fatigue, or for those who just needed some gentle exercise. In the five months since I've been taking the class I've learned to walk on the treadmill at three miles per hour for up to half an hour a day and to climb on the Stairmaster 14-15 flights at a time. These are things I never could do, even as a younger, stronger person. Regan has changed my life." ~ *Vicki*

"I feel energized! I feel great!" ~ *Sandy*

"This is the only program my doctor recommends and the only program I can do. I also enjoy it! I look forward to seeing Regan every week." ~*Willy*